HOW TO SURVIVE CANCER

A Plain Language Guide to Self-Coping

by

Ismail Kazem, MD, FACR, FASTRO

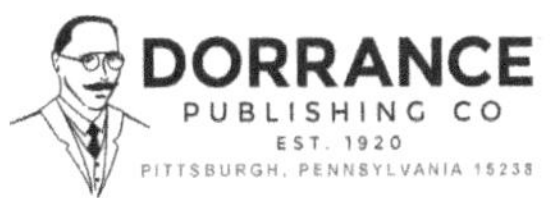

DORRANCE
PUBLISHING CO
EST. 1920
PITTSBURGH, PENNSYLVANIA 15238

Dorrance Publishing Co
585 Alpha Drive
Pittsburgh, PA 15238
Visit our website at *www.dorrancebookstore.com*

ISBN: 979-8-88729-305-9
eISBN: 979-8-88729-805-4

To my late brother,
Professor Mohamed Ibrahim Kazem,
God bless his soul.

He died of brain cancer, but his memory survives in our thoughts.

PREFACE

Life is a battle for survival. It begins with birth and ends in death. Between birth and death, one should enjoy a full life. Yet we are exposed every day of our being to innumerable risks: risks within our bodies, risks of our behavior, risks of our interaction with others, and risks of our environment.

We need to identify our risks to be able to reduce running into them. We also need to know our resources and our chances vis-a-vis running the risks. The most important health hazards in the USA other than accidents are heart disease and cancer.

This book is meant to be a road map in plain language to help those who are concerned about getting cancer so that they may confront the problem on a personal level in order for them to cope with their concerns successfully.

CONTENTS

PROLOGUE

"Fear builds its phantoms which are more fearsome than reality itself."

Jawaharlal Nehru

The evolution of the concept of surviving cancer across the epochs followed a path parallel to the advancement of human knowledge. About three thousand years BC, an Egyptian physician/priest described in a papyrus cases of tumors of the breast that he treated with a red-hot metal probe with poor outcome.

Medical history followed the rise and fall of nations and empires, and at each epoch, a wealth of information based on intelligent observation added to the wealth of human knowledge. For centuries, cancer as a disease was a taboo feared, whispered about, and considered hopeless. The Greek philosopher Hippocrates (460–377 BC), who is regarded as the father of medicine, advanced the idea that there are four basic elements that govern the universe: earth with quality of cold, air with dry, water with moist, and fire as hot. The human body likewise was governed by four fluids: blood, phlegm, yellow bile, and black bile. The four fluids must be in balance to maintain health. Disease resulted from any imbalance in these fluids. Cancer was thought to be the result of excessive production of black bile and incurable. Because of the appearance of the infiltration around the main tumor mass like the legs of a crab, Hippocrates coined the name cancer, *which is derived from the Greek word for crab. The lack of knowledge about cancer as a disease lingered for many centuries until the Renaissance, when scientific tools and reasoning became available. The concept of surviving cancer during the Dark Ages thus was irrelevant. Cancer was discovered in its advanced or end stages, and survival was only considered as a miracle that qualifies for sainthood. No wonder cancer was treated as a curse approached by prayers, superstitions, and faith. An example of the prevailing beliefs of the epoch is the legend of Saint Agatha, the patron saint of breast cancer. The story of Saint Agatha starts in the third century in the island of Sicily. She was from a noble family and possessed great beauty and charm. This tempted the Roman governor of Sicily to try to seduce her, but as a good Christian, she snubbed his advances. As punishment for her faith and chastity, he imprisoned her. When she continued to reject him, he became angry and ordered her breasts to be torn off her body with iron shears. And finally cast into a dungeon to die.*

Holding to her faith, she prayed the Lord to heal her wounds. She was visited by angels who comforted her, and in answer to her prayers, the miracle of restoring her breasts took place.

Across the centuries, important landmarks and milestones of new information and inventions enriched the medical knowledge and transformed it from art to science.

Thus, in 1590, a Dutch glassmaker invented the microscope. This rapidly paved the way in the 17th century for significant endeavors to research the human anatomy and physiology.

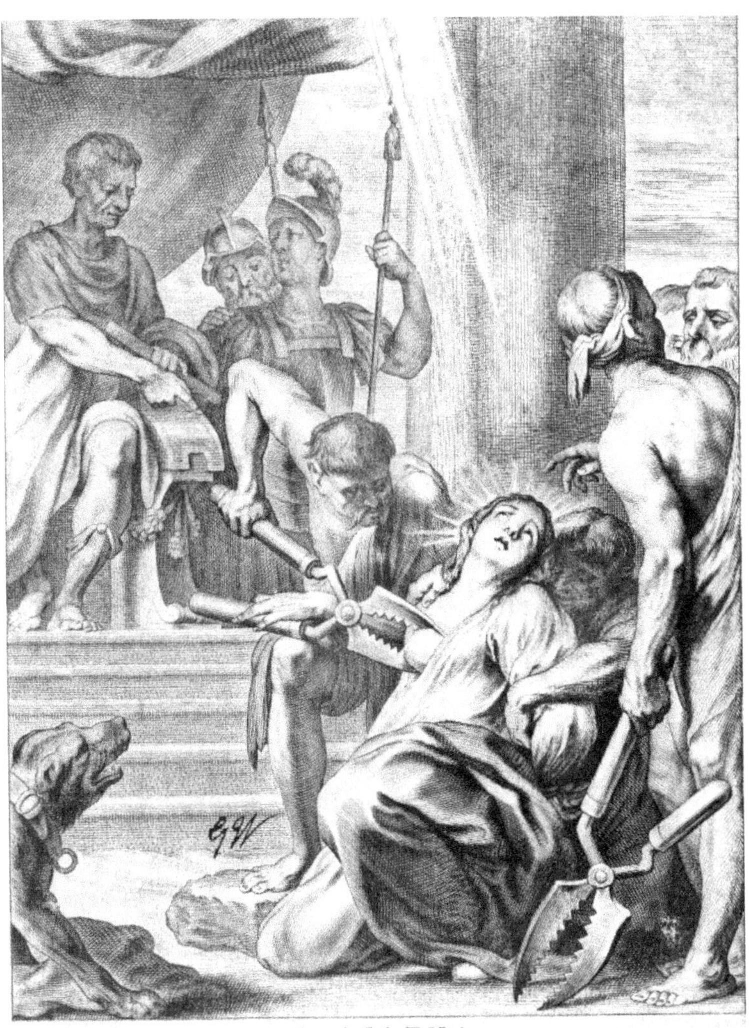

St. Agatha martyrdom, engraving mid-16th century.
(Welcome Collection).

Medical schools sponsored anatomy departments and taught human anatomy on dissected cadavers, which was previously banned.

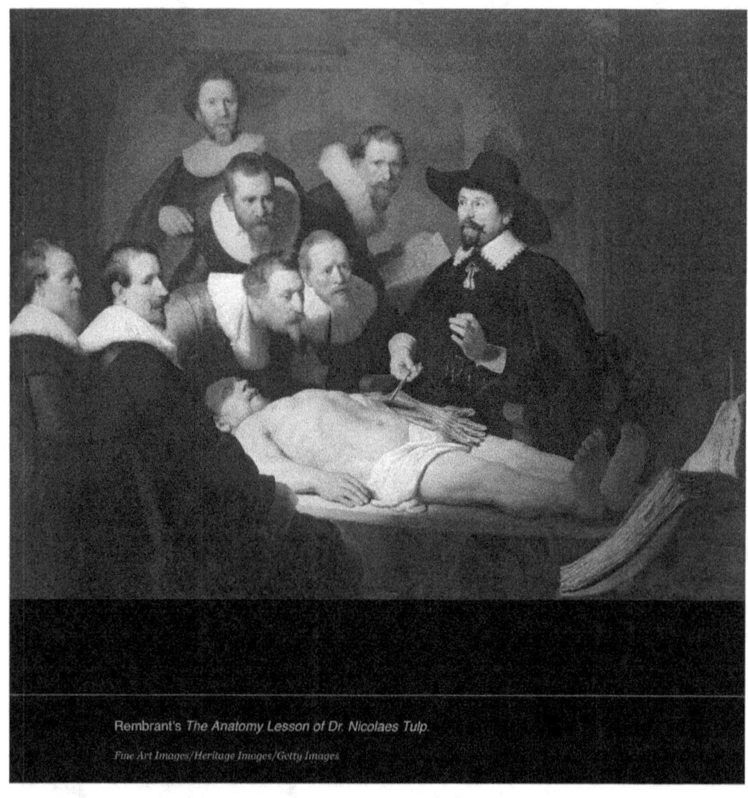

The Anatomy Lesson *was painted by Rembrandt in 1632.*

With anatomical knowledge and the availability of the micro- scope, the foundations of modern medicine were laid in the 17th century. Research in human anatomy, physiology and pathology be- came the focus of medical schools. The cancer cell was identified as different from the normal cell, and its spread through lymphatic vessels to lymph nodes was recognized. Surgical removal of cancer that was not fixed to its bed was attempted, but once the cancer was fixed or spread to lymph nodes, it was deemed untreatable. Research on what causes cancer and how to prevent it led Percival Pott, a British surgeon, to discover the relationship between cancer of the scrotum among chimney sweepers and their exposure to tar. This resulted in enacting a British law in 1788 to protect young boys working as chimney sweepers. Perhaps one of the first measures for cancer prevention.

In 1846 ether was introduced for anesthesia, and in 1866 Joseph Lister used carbolic acid sprays in the operating rooms for disinfection. These two events made it possible to perform surgery painlessly and improved its success by cutting down on wound infection.

By the end of the 19th century and beginning of the 20th century, major scientific discoveries took place and were instrumental in raising hopes for improving cancer survival.

The following landmark milestones were significant in understanding the nature of cancer and approaches to its treatment:

- *1895 Wilhelm Konrad Roentgen discovered X-rays, and in 1898 Marie and Pierre Curie isolated radium. Soon after, it was noted that both X-rays and radium radiations have biological effects on dividing cells. The treatment of cancer with X-rays and radium was thus applied initially with limited success, but eventually with improved technology and sophistication with great success.*

- *1911: A researcher named Peyton Rous found that a virus caused cancer in chickens. In 1915 a Japanese researcher named Yamagiwa induced cancer by applying coal tar to rabbit's ears.*

The same year, Alexis Carrel and Montrose Burrows pioneered tissue culture by growing cancer cells in laboratory flasks.

- *1928: George Papanicolau introduced the test known by his name (pap smear) for the detection of cancer of the uterus by examining cells obtained by a vaginal smear under the microscope.*
- *1937: President Franklin Roosevelt signed the creation of the National Cancer Institute to develop efficient ways to prevent, diagnose, and treat cancer.*
- *1953: James Watson, Francis Crick, and Maurice Wilkins shared a Nobel Prize for discovery of DNA structure. This started a new horizon in the genetic and molecular biology of cancer.*

In the past decades, new technologies and equipment were invented and utilized for improved diagnostic, imaging, and treatment of cancer, to mention a few: the CT (computer tomography), the linear accelerator, the MRI (magnetic resonance imaging), PET (positron emission tomography), PT (proton therapy)…etc. Novel chemotherapeutic agents, biopharmaceutics, evidence-based treatment protocols, and improved surgical and radiotherapy techniques have improved treatment outcome and reduced side effects.

The preceding review is a historical summary of the cancer problem that started as incurable and evolved into the achievement of curable survival. Yet despite all the progress, cancer, for some people, is a lingering taboo. Something not acceptable to say or mention. Fear and guilt prevent people from talking about cancer. Fear of pain and suffering and guilt or shame of having it. Being open about the issue and talking about it helps in seeking proper advice and increasing the chance for cure and survival. There are also several myths and misunderstandings about cancer. Only by talking about these openly can you dispel the apprehension. Cancer is not a death sentence. With early diagnosis and proper treatment, remission is achieved in most cases. Cancer is not contagious; therefore, there is no reason to avoid contact and socializing. Undergoing surgery or a biopsy does not cause cancer to spread. Exposure to cell phones, microwave ovens, or power lines are not proven to cause cancer. Herbal tea, natural food supplements, and diets neither cure nor prevent cancer.

Bottom line: Approach cancer with realistic acceptance. Do your best, expect the best, and accept the outcome. Seek and obtain help for coping as needed.

CHAPTER ONE

Surviving the Odds

*"Yea, though I walk through the valley of the shadow
of death, I fear no evil: for thou art with me."*

Psalm 23:4

According to the USA National Program of Cancer Registries, the probability of a person developing invasive cancer in one's life span that is from birth to death is one in three. In other words, a baby who is born today is confronted by a one-in-three chance that he or she would be diagnosed with cancer in his/her lifetime.

These odds, however, differ according to age-interval and gender. Thus, the odds for age interval from the time of birth till the age forty-nine years are one in thirty for men and one in eighteen for women. At age interval fifty to fifty-nine years, the odds for men and for women are the same at one in sixteen. At sixty to sixty-nine years of age, the odds for men are one in seven and for women one in ten. Above seventy years of age, the odds for men are one in 3 and for women one in four.

According to the National Center for Health Statistics, an estimated 1,806,590 new cancer cases and 606,520 deaths due to cancer were projected in the USA in the year 2020. Thanks to progress in cancer awareness, prevention efforts, early diagnosis, and improved treatment, a steady reduction in deaths due to cancer is noted since it peaked in 2017. An estimated 30 perccent fewer cancer deaths amount to approximately three million lives saved in this period.

Figures 1, 2, 3, and 4 represent ten leading cancer types for the estimated new cases and deaths according to gender in the USA in 2020.

On the individual level, the question is, What can be done to have the odds in one's favor?

First, what can be done to avoid having cancer, and if it cannot be prevented, what can be done to catch it early enough to have a better chance at cure?

A program for cancer prevention, screening, and early detection would thus have the following objectives:

- To reduce cancer incidence
- To reduce cancer mortality.
- To improve the quality of life for cancer survivors

To achieve these objectives let us first outline some definitions:

- Prevention: means to eliminate reverse or neutralize certain cancer-causing risk factors.

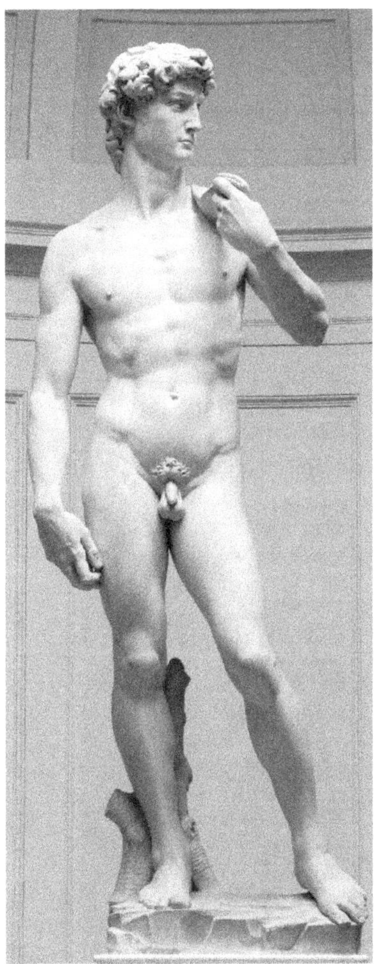

Figure 1: Estimated New Cancer Cases for Ten Leading Cancer Types in 2020 in Men

Prostate: 191,930	21%
Lung and Bronchus: 116,300	13%
Colon and Rectum: 78,300	9%
Urinary Bladder: 62,100	7%
Melanoma of the Skin: 60,190	7%
Kidney and Renal Pelvis: 45,520	5%
Non-Hodgkin lLymphoma: 42,380	5%
Oral Cavity and Pharynx: 38, 380	4%
Leukemia: 35,470	4%
Pancreas: 30,400	3%
All Sites: 893,660	100%

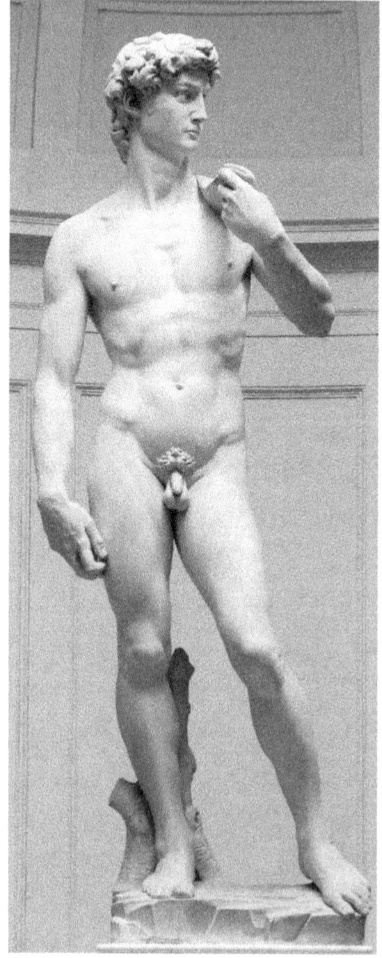

Figure 2: Estimated Cancer Deaths for Ten Leading Cancer Types in 2020 in Men

Lung and Bronchus: 72,500	23%
Prostate: 33,330	10%
Colon and Rectum: 28,630	9%
Pancreas: 24,640	8%
Liver and Bile Ducts: 20,020	6%
Leukemia: 13,420	4%
Esophagus: 13,100	4%
Urinary Bladder: 13,050	4%
Non-Hodgkin Lymphoma: 11,460	4%
Brain and Nervous System: 10,190	3%
All Sites: 321,160	100%

Estimates are rounded.

Source: USA Cancer Statistics 2020

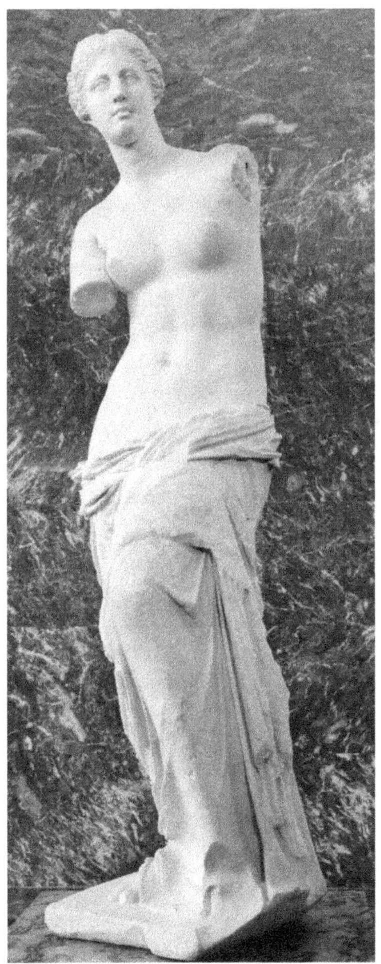

Figure 3: Estimated New Cancer Cases for Ten Leading Cancer Types in 2020 in Women

Breast: 276,480	30%
Lung and Bronchus: 112,520	12%
Colon and Rectum: 69,650	8%
Uterine Body: 65,620	7%
Thyroid: 40,170	4%
Melanoma of the Skin: 40,160	4%
Non-Hodgkin Lymphoma: 34,860	4%
Kidney and Renal Pelvis: 28,230	3%
Pancreas: 27,200	3%
Leukemia: 25,060	3%
All Sites: 912,930	100%

Estimates are rounded.

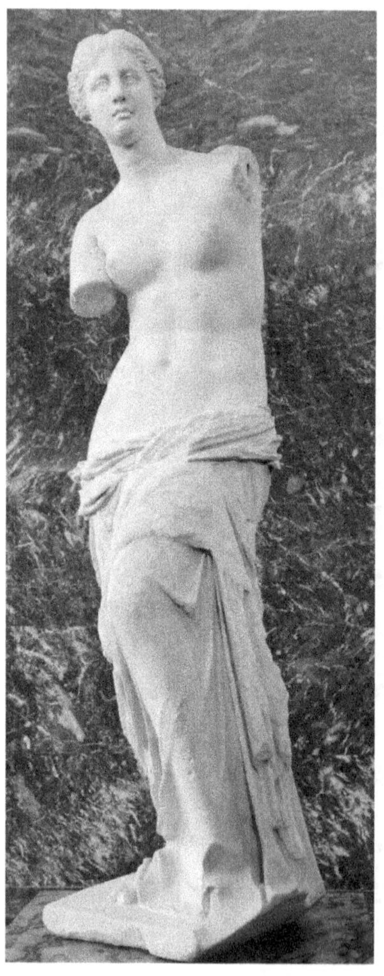

Figure 4: Estimate Cancer Deaths for Ten Leading Cancer Types in 2020 in Women

Lung and Bronchus: 63,220	22%
Breast: 42,170	15%
Colon and Rectum: 24,570	9%
Pancreas: 22,410	8%
Ovary: 13,940	5%
Body of the Uterus: 12,590	4%
Liver and Bile Ducts: 10,140	4%
Leukemia: 9,680	3%
Non-Hodgkin Lymphoma: 8,480	3%
Brain and Nervous System: 7,830	3%
All Sites: 285,360	100%

Source: USA Cancer Statistics 2020.

- Screening: means to test defined otherwise healthy people for signs of undeclared cancer.
- Early detection: means to be aware of early signs and symptoms of potential cancer presence for prompt clinical evaluation and tests to be able to find the cancer in early stage for early treatment.

To be able to put the discussion in perspective, let us explain what cancer is and what causes it.

Cancer is many diseases. They differ in cell type, aggressiveness, and outcome. However, they share one thing: cancer cells continue to grow and multiply regardless of the needs or well-being of the person harboring these cells. If not treated, it leads to the person's death. But what induces a normal cell to transform and grow wild to become cancer?

Several factors are identified that are known to cause cancer. These factors can work separately or together. Cancer is a multistage and multi-factorial process.

That means that more than one factor can be responsible for causing cancer.

A factor may initiate a change in a cell that would be influenced by other factors to go through several stages of the malignant transformation.

The following causes are identified as cancer-inducing factors:

Viruses

- HPV (Human Papilloma Virus). This is a group of viruses some of which are associated with cancer of the uterine cervix, anus, vagina, vulva, and penis. They are also associated with cancer of the mouth and throat. The virus is sexually transmitted. Fortunately, there is a vaccine that when given to girls and boys at age nine to twenty, it can give them immunity to prevent the infection.

- HV (Hepatitis B and C Viruses). Chronic infection of the liver with these viruses is linked to liver cancer. There is effective immunization against HBV, and there is effective treatment for HCV.

- HIV (Human Immunodeficiency Virus). This virus is sexually transmitted and can predispose to a type of skin cancer called Kaposi's sarcoma, anal cancer, Hodgkin's disease, cancer of the mouth and throat, and liver cancer.

- EBV (Epstein-Barr virus). This is a common virus that is spread by contact from person to person. It can cause mononucleosis or remain dormant without apparent symptoms. The infection is related to cancer of the nasopharynx and certain types of lymphomas.

- HTLV-1 (Human T-lymph trophic Virus-1). This virus is associated with lymphocytic leukemia and non-Hodgkin lymphoma. It is not common in the USA, but prevalent in Japan and South America and may be detected in USA immigrants.

Chemicals

There is a long list of chemicals that can directly or indirectly cause cancer. These can be in the environment due to pollution, or industrial with occupational exposures. Among these chemicals are chloroform, DDT, formaldehyde, and PCB (polychlorinated biphenyls). Environmental protection agencies and industrial safety regulations address these issues.

Physical Factors

This includes sunlight, heat, ionizing radiation (X-rays and gamma rays), and possibly electromagnetic power fields and microwaves.

Biological Factors

Genetic predisposition plays a role in cancer risk, as well as our hormonal status.

Lifestyle and Behavioral Factors

This includes what we eat and how much we eat, heavy alcohol consumption, smoking, inadequate health care for obesity, hypertension, and diabetes....For a normal cell to undergo transformation to a cancer cell, it goes through several sequence of events.

A normal cell has checks and balances that maintain its normal behavior for the body to remain healthy. This normal behavior is controlled by the cell's genetic material, which contains the instruction for its function. When the normal cell is exposed to a cancer-inducing agent, be it viral, chemical, or physical, certain molecules in the genetic material change. The change can be trivial, and the cell can repair it. Or it can be serious and disrupt its function. When the injured cell divides, it reproduces the changed genes; this change is called mutation. With every division, more transformation in the genetic material of mutated cells takes place, resulting in a cancer cell that has lost its normal checks and balances. With time, a tumor forms, and if not detected early enough, it becomes more aggressive and spreads elsewhere in the body. In the next page, a schematic representation illustrates the stages of cancer transformation and possible points of intervention.

PREVENTION

The most pressing question that we should confront is, Can cancer be prevented?

On a community scale, the answer is yes. On an individual level, the answer is it is possible to significantly reduce the chance of getting cancer.

Among successful cancer prevention measures are the following:

Community Education

Knowledge is the most effective means to combat fear. That is why the dissemination of information and facts about cancer is a public health priority. Public awareness of cancer risk factors and the way to deal with them can help in its prevention.

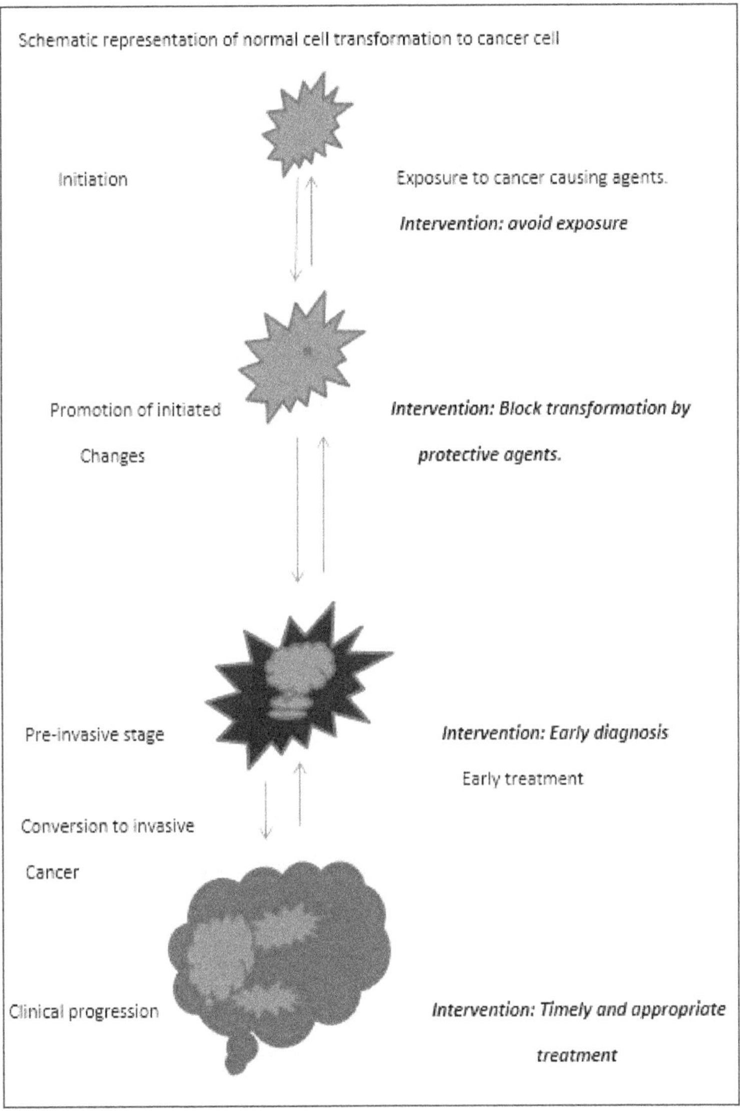

Schematic representation of normal cell transformation to cancer cell
Initiation
Exposure to cancer causing agents.
Intervention: avoid exposure
Promotion of initiated
Changes
Intervention: Block transformation by
protective agents.
Pre-invasive stage
Intervention: Early diagnosis
Early treatment
Conversion to invasive
Cancer
Clinical progression
Intervention: Timely and appropriate
treatment

Behavior Modification

The use of tobacco, whether by smoking or chewing, is proven to be associated with the risk of cancer of the lung, head and neck, esophagus and stomach, and bladder cancer. It is estimated that up to one of three cancer deaths in United States of America is caused by tobacco consumption.

Obviously, smoke cessation is a strong incentive in preventing cancer.

Excessive alcohol consumption is also associated with high risk for cancer of the mouth and of esophagus, cancer of the breast, and colorectal cancer.

Alcohol rehab programs contribute significantly to reducing the risk of cancer.

Promiscuity and unprotected sex are known risk factors for sexually transmitted infection and should be avoided to reduce the risk of cancer.

Immunization

As mentioned before, human papilloma virus infection is associated with the risk of cancer of the uterine cervix, vagina, anus, penis, and mouth and throat. Public awareness of the value of vaccination of boys and girls in their teens against HPV would reduce that risk.

Also, vaccination against Hepatitis B would reduce the risk of cancer of the liver.

Drug users are particularly at risk of infection with hepatitis C and HIV. Presently, there are no vaccines available to immunize against them. However, awareness of the role of needle sharing in transmitting the infection and needle exchange programs can help.

Radiation Exposure

Industrial and medical use of X-rays and gamma rays follows strict regulation to ensure the safety of users. Medical applications follow guidelines to avoid unnecessary tests and to reduce patients' exposure.

Brick-built homes are tested for radon gas, and if the level is above the permissible level, ventilation is required to dissipate the emanated gas.

Exposure to sunlight and ultraviolet radiation increases the risk of skin cancer, especially in fair-skinned people. Avoiding long exposure and use of sunscreens help reduce the risk.

Genetic and Family Counseling

A strong family history of cancer can indicate a genetic risk that requires further inquiry. A genetic counselor is the qualified person to effectively evaluate the risk and discuss the options of preventive intervention and their relevance to the individual's needs and choices.

Diet and Nutrition Counseling

The link between diet and cancer is rather vague and indirect. Whereas some studies showed a correlation between the incidence of cancer of the colon and red meat, lack of fiber, and high fat content, yet a cause and effect are hard to prove. A lot of social hype and misconception about diet and cancer unfortunately exists. Therefore, prudence and common sense should prevail. Bottom line: a healthy diet should include fruits, vegetables, low fat, high protein, and high fiber. However, it is not just a matter of quality but also quantity matters. Obesity and hypertension are strongly associated with cancer, as stated above. Thus, to reduce one's risk for cancer one needs a balanced diet along the lines mentioned. In addition, exercising, avoiding overweight, avoiding smoking and excessive alcohol consumption.

Chemo Protection

Persons that are identified as having high risk factors for certain cancers either by virtue of genetic predisposition, presence of premalignant condition, or known behavior lifestyle may benefit from the administration of certain medications that can prevent cancer.

For example, it is known that some breast cancers feed on the female hormone estrogen. Women with strong family predisposition to breast cancer may therefore benefit from the administration of medications that suppress the production of estrogen such as Tamoxifen or Raloxifene.

Similarly, prostate cancer depends on the male hormone for its growth. The administration of a drug that neutralizes the production of the male hormone like Finasteride may help reduce the risk of cancer of the prostate.

Recently, Aspirin was recognized as a player in reducing the risk of cancer of the colon and is frequently included in the management of persons with high risk for colorectal cancer.

Several vitamins and food supplements like vitamin B12, B6, C, E, A, D, and selenium have been proposed to lower the risk of cancer either as direct benefit or to presumably improve the immune response. Unfortunately, there is no hard evidence in support of such claims.

SCREENING PROGRAMS

As mentioned above, screening means to test a defined group of otherwise healthy people for signs of undeclared cancer. Based on evidence and experience, guidelines for different body sites are developed on the one hand to minimize inconvenience and on the other hand to be cost effective.

The US Preventive Services Task Force is an independent volunteer panel of national experts in disease prevention and evidence-based medicine. The Task Force works to improve the health of all Americans by making evidence-based recommendations about clinical preventive services. Your primary care provider utilizes these guidelines to decide on who would benefit most from which screening test according to gender and age group. Examples of these guidelines are listed below.

Breast Cancer Screening
- Breast self-examination by women twenty years and older.
- Examination of the breasts by a health care professional every three years from age twenty to forty, then annually.
- Optional Base line mammogram at age forty and every two years.

- Recommended screening mammogram every two years for women aged fifty to seventy-four years.

Uterine Screening

- Screening with cervical cytology (pap smear) is recommended for sexually active women from age twenty-one and every three years until age sixty-five.
- Testing for HPV infection is also considered.
- Base line endometrial biopsy for high-risk women, i.e., with history of infertility, obesity, hypertension, diabetes, or hormone therapy.

Colon and Rectal Screening

- Digital rectal exam every year after age forty.
- Stool blood test every year after age forty-five.
- Sigmoidoscopy every –three to five years after age forty-five.

Prostate Screening

There have been lately ongoing discussions about the merits of subjecting low-risk men for routine prostate cancer screening with PSA (prostate specific antigen) test. A moderate approach includes the following:

- Men forty years and older should have a digital rectal exam annually as part of general medical checkup. If an enlarged prostate or a nodule is felt by the clinician, further appropriate evaluation would be justified.

- For men –fifty to sixty-five years of age, a base line PSA test is suggested, if normal annual testing is optional.

As a rule, one should recognize that the most common cancer risk factors are:

- *Current tobacco use.*
- *Chronic alcohol consumption.*
- *Overweight.*
- *Poor health care maintenance, neglected diabetes, hypertension, etc.*
- *Strong family history of cancer.*

<u>EARLY DETECTION</u>

One cannot over emphasize the fact that treating cancer in its early stages offers the best chance not only for cure but also for the best quality of life. It is therefore important to recognize the early warning signs that should prompt immediate attention and appropriate medical examination. Ignoring these signs may lead to a delay in detecting early cancer and fore sake the opportunity of effective early treatment.

The following are the most common warning signs that warrant attention:

- Changes in bowel habits
- Changes in urination
- A sore that does not heal promptly
- Unusual bleeding or discharge

- A lump or thickening of tissues
- Indigestion or trouble swallowing
- Recent change in size or appearance of a wart, mole, or new skin changes
- Nagging cough or hoarseness of voice
- Other non-specific signs include unexplained weight loss, chronic fatigue, persistent pain, and fever of unknown origin.

It should be realized that annual medical examination is an important part of early detection.

Your medical provider is trained to recognize and evaluate abnormal signs and symptoms that may trigger concern. If necessary, blood tests or imaging tests can be ordered, and timely referral to the appropriate specialist can be made.

CHAPTER TWO:

The First Encounter

For now, we see through a glass darkly!

Corinthians 13:12

The management of cancer is a process that begins by a visit to your primary care physician. Clinical evaluation would start by a good history that includes among other things:

- Duration of symptoms
- Possible causative or risk factors
- Possible underlying chronic disease
- Family history, including close relatives, parents, and siblings

This is followed by a thorough physical exam that includes systematic site evaluation with special attention to regional lymph nodes. Evaluation for enlarged organs, skin ulceration, nodularity, change in consistency, swelling, bleeding, discharge, tenderness, or lumps.

Based on the findings of the physical exam, relevant work up is ordered. This may include endoscopy, imaging (X-rays, CT scans, MRI, US, nuclear imaging).

Laboratory tests including blood counts, blood chemistry, hormone profile, tumor markers,…etc.

Once the results are reported and reviewed, consideration for tissue diagnosis is made by obtaining a biopsy. If possible, this can be obtained by inserting a needle in the suspected growth and retrieving enough cells or tissues to make the diagnosis under the microscope. Often the needle must be guided by ultrasound imaging, CT imaging, or MRI imaging. For deeply seated tumors, it may be necessary to arrange for the examination under general anesthesia.

The sample of tissues thus obtained is sent to the pathology lab for processing with specific substances to help identify the type of cancer under the microscope. The pathology report would not only describe the type of cancer cells but also its degree of aggressiveness. If relevant, special processing of the biopsy tissue is made to obtain additional information about the characteristic of the tumor, e.g., whether it has certain affinity to a specific hormone or a specific genetic marker that would help in the choice of treatment.

Once the type of cancer is identified, a medical oncologist is consulted and additional work-up tests are considered to determine the extent of the tumor. This process is called staging work up. It consists of surveying the body with imaging for evidence of spread to lymph nodes, bone, or internal organs. Accordingly, the stage of the cancer is mapped and sorted out as to size of the primary tumor, presence or absence of lymph node spread, and presence or absence of distant spread to bone or organs.

The resulting information is tabulated as T (tumor) N (lymph nodes) M (metastases) stage.

The plan of treatment is determined by identifying the cell type and its aggressiveness, i.e., its grade, and the TNM stage, i.e., its extent.

Usually, three grades are identified by the pathologist:

- low grade
- intermediate grade
- high grade

Depending on how the malignant cells bear similarity to the benign cell of origin, presence, or absence of invasion of surrounding tissue, lymph vessels, or blood vessels.

Four stages are also identified based on the size of the tumor and presence or absence of regional or distant spread.

Generally speaking,

- Stage I is a tumor measuring two centimeters or less with no spread to regional nodes or elsewhere.
- Stage II is when the tumor measures –three to five centimeters or with spread to less than two regional lymph nodes.
- Stage III is when the tumor measures more than five centimeters or has spread to more than three regional lymph nodes.

- Stage IV is when evidence of distant spread of the cancer is established.

This is a rough description of the designation of the stage of the cancer. It should be realized that there is a more refined stage description for each cancer type.

The diagnosis and management of cancer is a teamwork involving several cancer specialists and medical professionals. This is because cancer can be treated in different ways depending on the cell type, degree of aggressiveness, i.e., its grade, and its extent, i.e., stage. The treatment can be by surgery, radiation therapy, chemotherapy, immunotherapy, or combination of one or all of these. In most cancer centers, the treatment and management of every new patient diagnosed with cancer is discussed by a committee called the tumor board or cancer committee. The committee includes a general radiologist, interventional radiologist, pathologist, cancer surgeon, medical oncologist, radiation oncologist, oncology nurse, social worker, and occupational therapist if relevant. During the meeting of such a committee, all information pertaining to every new patient is reviewed and discussed. If additional tests or consultations are needed, they would be proposed. When all of the patient's evaluation is complete, the best line of treatment is agreed upon. Usually evidence-based guidelines and accepted peer-reviewed treatment protocols are applied for decision making. This way the best available treatment or treatment options are obtained, documented, and shared with the treating oncologist to be discussed with the patient. Appointments are accordingly made with the relevant service or specialist.

CHAPTER THREE:
Let Us Talk

"Ask and it shall be given you, seek and ye shall find, knock and it shall be opened unto you."

Matthew 7:7

After the completion of diagnostic and staging work-up, your oncologist will schedule an appointment to go over the results and discuss the treatment options. It is prudent that before you go that you would do some research about your type of cancer and the available treatment modalities, how they work, and how they relate to one another. Be prepared both to ask questions and to answer questions. Know your rights in terms of insurance-covered expenses and sick leave if needed. Secure a support system whether by family members, friends, or caregivers. Be assertive and confront your fears by having faith in your resilience and inner strength. When you go for your appointment, have a family member or friend accompany you. You may misunderstand or forget the information discussed, so your companion can remind you or facilitate your understanding. Remember that you are not just a patient, you are, above all, a PERSON. You are entitled to maximize your wellbeing.

As mentioned before, cancer is treated by several modalities either alone or in combination depending on the cancer type and extent. The role of each type of treatment is discussed below:

Surgery

Surgery may be needed to obtain a diagnostic biopsy. But it is also an amazingly effective modality of treatment. It may be limited to removing the tumor, removing a part of whole organ, or removal of a whole organ, and associated regional lymph nodes. What determines the type and extent of the surgery is the type and extent of the cancer as well as the resulting status of functionality and cosmesis for the patient. For example, surgery for brain cancer is limited in extent to avoid drastic loss of function. The cancer surgeon attempts as much as possible to preserve an organ if this does not jeopardize the chance of cure. For example, a small cancer in the female breast may be removed with a safe margin preserving the rest of the breast for post-operative radiation treatment, chemotherapy, and/or hormone treatments as appropriate.

In summary, the extent of surgery is not only guided by the type and extent of the cancer but also by an attempt to avoid mutilation, loss of function, and serious complications. However, there are situations when extensive surgery is needed. In these cases, the defect left after the removal of the cancer-bearing tissues is repaired by reconstructive surgery using the patient's skin or muscle grafts.

There are modern surgical techniques that improve the outcome and, in some cases, speed up the recovery and shorten hospital stays. These techniques use robotic computer assistance and a small access incision.

When you are seen by the surgeon, the findings of the evaluation and tests will be once again reviewed, and the reason for the surgery will be discussed as well as the type of procedure planned. The potential side effects and chance for complications will be explained. The surgeon may use a diagram or picture or a model to help explain the anatomy and the part of the body involved in the procedure. This information is usually reinforced by the surgical nurse, and frequently, some literature brochures are given with explanations and instructions.

Before you go for surgery you meet the anesthesiologist who will examine you to make sure you have no health issues that require special attention to avoid heart or breathing problems during the surgery. A blood sample is obtained to know your blood type to be matched if blood transfusion is needed during the surgery. After the completion of the surgery, you are escorted to the recovery room for observation, and once the condition is stabilized, you go to the appropriate nursing station unless it was a minor surgery and you can go home.

Before you go home you will be scheduled for follow-up appointments about a week to two weeks after the surgery to monitor the healing and remove the stitches if relevant. You will also be scheduled to see the medical oncologist or the radiation oncologist according to the management plan.

Surgery has also a role to play in palliative management of cancer. For example, relieving bowel obstruction, or relieving biliary obstruction by removing the reason for the blockage or by creating an artificial opening or passage to maintain the required flow. Post-operative care depends on the type and extent of the surgery. It can be brief, limited to removal of the stitches and monitoring prompt wound healing. But it can be lengthy and protracted. Rehabilitation and occupational therapy may be needed. Managing of muscle weakness or extremity swelling resulting from the surgery would need skilled professionals. If an organ or a limb is surgically removed, appropriate prosthesis or reconstructive procedure would be needed. If the voice box must be removed, for example, a voice prosthesis can be provided, and the patient would need to be educated on how to care for the air opening in the neck, called tracheostoma. Patients left with a bowel opening or stomach opening, colostomy, or gastrostomy would also be educated about the care of their stoma.

Radiation Treatments

Radiation therapy can be used as the sole treatment modality or in combination with surgery and/or chemotherapy and immunotherapy. It is used for the definitive treatment of some early cancer sites with curative intent, as adjuvant to other treatment modalities to enhance the probability of cures, or to improve local disease control. It is also used in advanced disease for relieving of symptoms such as pain, relief of pressure on critical organs, or to stop bleeding due to tumor ulceration. In the past century, radiation oncology reached a high degree of sophistication. High energy X-rays and some atomic particles can be beamed with precision to the part of the body that harbors the cancer cells. Radioactive sources can also be implanted in the tumor-bearing organ to deliver the radiation energy directly to the cancer. The radiation, when absorbed by the cancer-bearing tissues, induces chemical changes in the nucleus of cancer cells, which disrupts their ability to divide. The inactivated cancer cells wither and die and are eliminated from the body.

With precise technology, 3-D treatment planning based on accurate imaging and better understanding of tumor lethal dose and normal tissue tolerance, more cures, and fewer side effects are attainable. Computer and space technologies have impacted all aspects of medical practice, and radiation oncology has benefited tremendously.

High-energy linear accelerators and proton-beam radiation units are now available relatively compact in size but highly sophisticated in performance. Precision movement of the treatment table and radiation beam can be programmed and automated. The energy levels of the radiation beams can be selected as appropriate. The shape of the treatment field can be designed to conform with the desired contour of the target volume. Thermoplastics and various immobilization molds and devices help support the patient in position for accurate reproduction during daily treatment sessions.

The introduction of CT-based and MRI-based tumor localization and treatment simulation eliminated the guesswork from radiation treatment planning. The radiation oncology simulator provides CT-image slices of the body, which are digitally reconstructed to provide accurate outline of the body contour, definition of anatomic boundaries, and delineation of the tumor target volume as well as nearby critical organs that need to be protected and spared damaging radiation. 3-D rendition allows 3-D conformal radiation treatment planning. Treatment planning programs provide radiation dose distribution in the selected target volumes. Thus, the radiation oncologist can determine immediately region of under or over dosage within the total volume. By varying the amount of radiation provided by each beam, optimum distribution can be achieved. A sophisticated program allows what is called inverse planning. This allows the radiation physics team and the radiation oncologist to plot the desired ideal dose distribution, and the computer program determines the intensity and direction of the needed radiation beams.

A special application called stereo-tactic radiosurgery is applied to treat small tumor volumes with a high radiation dose. This can be used for example in treating a small brain tumor close to vital part of the brain where surgery would be too risky, or other parts of the body when a patient's condition does not allow safe surgical procedure.

Radiation treatments use imposing equipment that can seem overwhelming or even threatening. Immobilization devises are used to avoid movement during the treatment that usually lasts few minutes. During the treatment, patients are placed comfortably on the treatment couch with the immobilization devices and left alone in the treatment vault. However, they are continuously monitored by the treating therapist through video and audio contact. Any sign of distress or discomfort is immediately attended to. Patients who suffer from claustrophobia are assured and encouraged. Relaxing music may be provided, and in extreme cases, if needed, a tranquilizer is administered.

In addition to external beam radiation treatments, radiation sources can be inserted in body cavities or implanted in cancerous tissues. Such techniques are called brachytherapy, meaning *short-distance treatment*. Depending on the situation, local or general anesthesia is administered.

Chemotherapy

As mentioned before, cancer surgery and radiation treatments deal with local and regional spread of cancer, while chemotherapy has a systemic effect through its blood distribution, reaching all over the body.

Cancer chemotherapy employs many chemical compounds that exert harmful effects on dividing cells. This results in interference with the cell's ability to reproduce or inducing a degree of toxicity that leads to the death of the cell.

The chemotherapeutic agents are usually administered by intravenous infusion, intramuscular injections, or by mouth in the form of tablets or capsules.

For tumors that are sensitive and susceptible to chemotherapeutic agents like leukemia and lymphoma, the treatment can have curative intent. In other situations, the treatment objective can be one or more of the following:

- <u>Neoadjuvant:</u> That is given before surgery and/or radiation therapy.

- <u>Adjuvant:</u> That is given along radiation treatments either concurrently or at intervals after surgery or radiation therapy.
- <u>Palliative:</u> In situations where the disease is advanced but the objective is to slow its progression or improve the patient's condition.

Historically, cancer was treated by toxic chemicals administered in small gradual doses that included compounds of mercury, lead, sulfur, iron, copper, arsenic, iodine, and potassium. Modern chemotherapy was ushered by an incident during the Second World War. On December 3rd, 1943, the USS *Liberty* was docked in Bari, Italy, when it was targeted by German fire. The *Liberty* carried a cargo of several barrels of nitrogen mustard gas, secretly intended for chemical warfare. Many sailors were killed by the leaked gas. Those who survived suffered a significant decrease in their white cell count. This observation led to the idea of exploring mustard gas as a treatment for leukemia, a cancer of the blood white cells. Further research showed that mustard gas can stop the division of some cancer cells.

Since that time, cancer research provided many chemotherapeutic agents that showed great success in treating different types of cancer. Some are called cytotoxic, meaning that they poison the dividing cell, causing its death, and some are called cytostatic, meaning that they stop the cell from dividing.

The cancer cell goes through a cycle from a resting cell to a metabolically active phase, during which it manufactures enough molecules to double the nuclear material before it enters the division phase. Some chemotherapy agents are cell cycle-specific agents, others are independent of the cell cycle, meaning they can inactivate the cancer cell regardless of its phase of development.

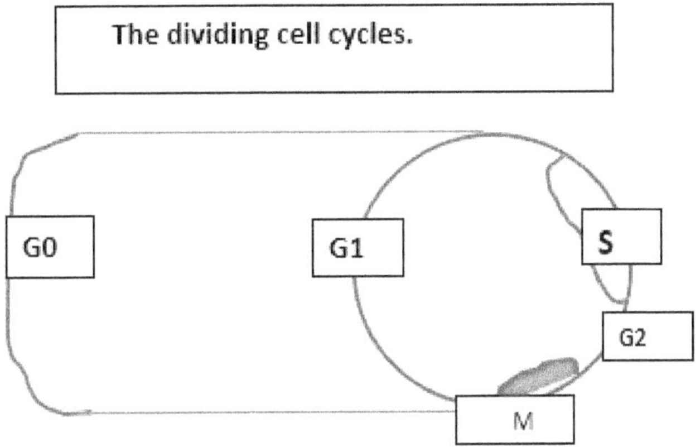

G0: resting phase. The cell is inactive.

G1: Interval between cell division and synthesis.

S: DNA synthesis phase.

G2: interval for turning DNA into chromosomes.

M: cell division phase.

In treating a person with cancer, more than one chemotherapeutic agent is used. This way the treatment can combine different mechanisms of action to optimize the effect on the cancer and minimize the side effects. The combined drugs are usually administered in cycles varying from a week to several weeks according to a schedule planned beforehand and discussed with the person receiving the treatment. The course of treatment can vary from six to twelve cycles depending on the type and stage of the cancer. The strategy of treatment is usually started by induction, meaning priming the cancer for response, followed by consolidation of the response. If the response is suboptimal, intensification of the treatment is considered either by increasing the dose or adding another agent. Following the achievement of a clinical response continuation of the treatment may be considered for consolidation of the achieved response or for maintaining a hold on the cancer to stop it from recurrence.

Biologic Response Modifiers and Immunotherapy

Biologic response modifiers are therapeutic agents that alter the interaction of the host, meaning the person, and the cancer.

The human body is not immune to the risk of disease, but it is endowed by a sophisticated defense mechanism that can fend against exposure to harmful external or internal foreign agents. The immune system is one of the defense mechanisms that the body uses to stop infection and to neutralize alien proteins that the body recognizes as unhealthy. There are two ways that the immune system responds with to combat or neutralize unwanted infection: 1. The first with antibodies that are naturally available or acquired in response to a challenging protein. These antibodies are produced by specialized white cells called B-lymphocytes, and the challenging protein is called an antigen. Thus, the antibodies combine with the antigen and neutralize it. 2. The second is to launch activated killer cells called

T-lymphocytes that attack the offending antigen by swallowing and dissolving it using appropriate enzymes.

Cancer cells are not recognized by the body as normal and thus considered as alien protein. In the early development of the cancer with few cells, the immune system can cope with the challenge and use antibodies and killer cells to arrest its growth. But as the tumor grows beyond the ability of the immune system, it continues to progress and spread.

Advances in cancer research identified the biology of the cancer cell and its interaction with the immune system. This paved the way for developing strategies that can modify the immune response of the body towards the cancer by applying a class of pharmaceuticals called biologic response modifiers, or immunotherapeutic. These biologic agents include the use of specific antibodies, enzymes that arrest cancer growth called cytokines, specialized cells called tumor necrosis factor...etc.

These biologics work through:

- direct toxic effect on tumor cells,
- restoring or strengthening or modifying tumor-immune response,
- modifying other biologic effects by interfering with tumor cell metabolism, ability to spread and metastasize.

Biotherapy can thus be active or passive, specific, or nonspecific.

Active: substances that induce direct effect through immunization, like vaccines.

Passive: agents that boost the immune system.

Biotherapy is usually combined with chemotherapy to enhance its effect. But recently the use of biotherapy is recognized as effective front-line treatment for certain types of cancer. It is now possible to analyze the genetic composition of the tumor whereby the characteristics of the cancer cell are identified to help in the prediction of its vulnerability to a specific biologic or chemotherapeutic agent.

Currently, more promising agents are in the pipeline that hopefully will be more effective with less side effects. The future holds exciting possibilities for targeting the cancer cell with appropriate agents that kill cancer while sparing the normal tissues!

BUT BEWARE OF TREATMENT FRAUD: The treatments outlined above are scientifically developed and based on clinical evidence; unfortunately, however, there are charlatans and quacks who take advantage of innocent and trusting patients offering promising "cures" that may be harmful, and if not, they would at least delay effective treatments. Confronted with the initial diagnosis or a recurrence of cancer, some patients feel threatened and remorseful. Without support and assurance of their treating oncologist, they may seek "alternative" ineffective treatment. It is therefore important to be aware of such disproven treatments and expose the fraud committed by the quacks who offer them.

Unproven Cancer Treatments

Patients diagnosed with cancer can be vulnerable to offers of "miracle" cures. Claims of bogus treatments that are natural, nutritional, to strengthen the immune system, or as cure-all should be critically scrutinized, researched, and questioned.

Shady cancer clinics in this country and abroad, mostly in Mexico, try to lure their victims. They promote fanciful theories of the causes of cancer and pretend to neutralize them claiming that their ineffective treatments are soundly based. Access to social media and online advertisements are facilitating the spread of cancer treatment scams under the guise of alternative or "natural" treatments for cancer "cures." Friends and well-wishers unwittingly can pass on misinformation in a misguided attempt to be helpful. The Federal Trade Commission (consumer.ftc.gov) is one of several resources on the web to check out these scams. Other resources include cancer.gov, nih.gov, Americancancersociety.org, and several reputable cancer centers.

A very useful outline of alternative treatments that have been promoted to treat or prevent cancer but lack scientific and medical evidence of effectiveness can be found on "en.wikipedia.org." It lists unproven and disproven cancer treatments with extensive evidence-based references.

CHAPTER FOUR:
Staying the Course

"Let us learn to appreciate there will be times when the trees will be bare, and look forward to the time when we may pick the fruit."

Anton Chekhov

In the previous chapter the different ways of treating cancer were described. The how and why they are used. In this chapter, I want to walk along with you as you receive the treatment. Consider the treatment as a journey and expect its ups and downs. Be grateful for the ups and persevere for the downs.

Whether surgery, radiation, chemotherapy, or immune therapy, each and all will task you physically and mentally. You can mostly cope with all the stress and side effects with the help of your oncologist and oncology nurse. But you may also need your own support system, be it your spouse, your family, or your friends. If need be, get help from your social worker or a help-group. Whatever the downs, stay the course and do not quit; the sun will shine after the storm.

At the start, the plan of your treatment was explained and discussed with your oncologist, but going through the journey is a different experience. Unless you were treated for an exceedingly early cancer that can be completely removed surgically, a treatment plan takes anywhere from six months to a year, and in certain cases longer. During this time, you will undergo periodical clinical re-evaluation, blood tests, and imaging as needed. Based on the re-evaluation and interim tests, modifications of the treatment plan may be necessary.

Most of the side effects of the treatments are successfully managed by medications that may be administered preemptively or symptomatically, for example to treat nausea, diarrhea, lack of appetite, pain, or discomfort. Radiation treatments may cause skin irritation or even burn. This would be monitored by your radiation oncologist and appropriate lotions and ointments will be given to lessen the discomfort and promote the healing. While treating head and neck cancer, or lung cancer with combined chemotherapy and radiation therapy, sometimes the lining of the mouth, throat, and esophagus becomes intensely irritated such that eating and swallowing can become very painful. A feeding tube may be necessary in this situation to maintain adequate nourishment. Most chemotherapeutic agents are given as intravenous infusion. To facilitate their administration, a special catheter is implanted in a vein in the upper chest called porta-cath. To avoid its being blocked by blood clots, it is periodically flushed to keep it open. During a course of chemotherapy, the white blood cell count may fall; this requires modification of the dose or timing of the chemotherapy agents. If the count is significantly low, a specific drug called colony stimulating factor is given to stimulate the bone marrow to produce more while cells. In some cases, a blood transfusion may be necessary to make sure the body has adequate oxygenation.

The guidance of the oncologist and the oncology nurse and their monitoring of the treated person's condition and the response to treatment encourages the patient in surmounting the side effects.

One of the major concerns for female patients is the loss of hair after chemotherapy. This concern can be temporarily addressed by securing a wig or a head scarf. Reassurance that the hair will grow back after recovery makes it acceptable. Another concern for younger patients is the effect on menstruation and fertility. A consultation with a gynecologist can address this concern. For men, there could be concern about erectile dysfunction, and for the younger ones about sterility. Counseling by a urologist about collecting and freeze-storing of sperm would ease the patient's mind. The possibility of erectile dysfunction needs to be addressed as well.

However, sometimes additional help may be needed. A dietitian can be consulted on feeding and nutritional advise. The social worker can be of help in facilitating some of the necessary logistics of finances, transportation, or domestic situations.

The treatment experience can be stressful and sometimes depressive. A support system at home can also be stressed. A psychologist intervention may be necessary to counsel the patient and family. Such intervention can be invaluable in bringing hope and positive outlook to the patient and family. In addition, there are several support groups that can be very helpful. They can help you feel better and more hopeful. They would allow you to talk about your feelings and deal with practical issues. Such support groups are meetings of people with cancer or have been in one way or another involved with cancer.

Some of these groups are devoted to one type of cancer, like breast cancer or lung or prostate etc., or suited to certain age group, gender, culture, or faith. They may meet online or in person. Some are sponsored by cancer organizations, and some are private. The American Cancer Society, the National Cancer Institute, and the CDC are some of the resources that can be reached for information and guidance about such groups.

Practicing relaxation exercises such as yoga and light sport activities is also helpful in promoting motivation and a sense of well-being.

Hope is the most important factor in surmounting the hardship of the treatment. One should remember that all the side effects and the stress of the treatment will eventually heal. At the end of it all, what counts is the hope for being healed and healthy once again.

CHAPTER FIVE:
Then What?

"Don't count the days, make the days count."
Mohamed Ali

The completion of a treatment plan is the end of a journey and the start of another. What follows depends on the objective of the treatment plan whether with the intention to cure the cancer or to arrest it or to palliate certain symptoms. A follow-up plan is thus formulated. The purpose of which is to assess the outcome of the treatment, manage any lingering side effects, detect any complications of the treatment, and be on the lookout for cancer re-activation to be able to treat it in time.

For early cancers, treatment plans aim for cure. The follow-up schedule is usually a month after the completion of the treatment, then six weeks to two months afterwards, then three, six and twelve months thereafter. If the treated person remains cancer free, annual follow-ups would be scheduled almost indefinitely.

During the follow-up visits, in addition to clinical evaluation of the patient as a whole and the status of the cancer, blood and imaging tests are also requested for the thorough assessment of the cancer status.

The results of the evaluations define the outcome of the treatment.

This outcome can be described in several ways that need to be defined:

- Remission: meaning complete response and absence of detectable disease.
- Incomplete or partial response: meaning some reduction of measurable disease but there is residual tumor, locally, regionally, or metastatic.
- No response: meaning the disease has progressed.
- Cure: means that the treated person remains cancer free for more than twenty years.

One should realize that, unfortunately, cancer recurrence after twenty years, though exceedingly rare, can happen. One should also remember that a person cured of one type of cancer may develop another type of cancer later. Hence a keen follow-up evaluation is necessary.

Following the completion of the treatment plan and before the scheduled follow-up examination there is a period of potential anxiety.

During the treatment, time is organized and structured. The daily or weekly interaction with the treatment team offers support and assurance. Being left with time in-between follow ups can leave you with a sort of vacuum. That is why you should get busy and productive. Set your mind on a quality time. Think positively and enjoy life. If you are employed, go back to work, whether part or full time according to your ability. Be social and enjoy your family. If you need to increase your physical performance, go to the gym or consult a physiotherapist. Make sure you eat healthy food and avoid over-eating or going hungry.

Time is your friend; do not make it your enemy. By that I mean do not dwell on uncertainty, rather have a positive outlook. If you feel comfortable, be confident and trust your body. When you go for your scheduled follow-up appointment, do not be intimidated by anticipation. Learn how to expect good news. Celebrate your wellness and acknowledge victory when asked by friends how you are doing.

Make your scheduled follow-up examination an opportunity to confirm that you are doing well. In between of these visits, be alert of any persistent unusual sensation, discomfort, or body changes. Report your concerns to your oncologist for reassurance about its significance. Schedule an earlier appointment if necessary.

If you have recovered and are in remission, feel blessed and be cheerful.

CHAPTER SIX:
What If?

"Success is not final; failure is not fatal: it is the courage to continue that counts."

Winston Churchill

The news of a recurrent cancer can be a devastating disappointment. Do not panic. Cancer is a chronic disease, and with appropriate management it can be controlled or arrested. If on a follow-up examination your oncologist finds out that the cancer has recurred, complete evaluation of the status of the cancer will be made. This is called "re-staging"; it is an assessment of the extent of the recurrence, whether it is local, regional, or widespread. Depending on this evaluation, a second line of treatment will be offered. You should discuss the situation and ask about the intensity of the treatment, outcome expectation, and potential side effects.

The re-staging process involves blood and imaging tests. Sometimes a needle biopsy is requested to confirm the recurrence and to evaluate the cancer cells for signs of change in their aggressiveness.

If the recurrence is deemed local, a limited surgical excision may be considered, followed by consolidation radiation or chemotherapy.

If on the other hand the cancer is found to have progressed, appropriate systemic chemotherapy and/or immune therapy will be offered.

Recurrent cancer may be discovered after a short or long period of declared remission. The intensity of second-line treatment depends on the patient's general condition, age, associated disease such as diabetes, hypertension, and heart disease. Achieving a remission after a recurrence is possible. That is why patients in good physical condition should be motivated to go ahead with second-line treatment. Even if complete response and remission is not achieved, the benefits of arresting the progress of the cancer and improving its symptoms is worthwhile.

Patients receiving second-line treatment require special support system. First, they must overcome the disappointment of the recurrence of the cancer. Second, they must be motivated to undergo second-line treatment. Third, they must tolerate and cope with the side effects of the treatment.

Collective counseling efforts by the oncologist, oncology nurse, and social worker in explaining the situation are essential. Family and friends' support are of great help. Understanding the individual reaction of the patient is needed. Some would feel angry and betrayed after hoping for the cure. Some may lose confidence in the treatment and the treating team. Offering the possibility of a second opinion can help in regaining the confidence. Support groups and group therapy can be highly effective for the patient feeling not alone in the predicament of the recurrence.

As the second-line treatment proceeds, patients usually feel encouraged and accept the situation. Hope would raise their morale as they anticipate a second chance.

After the completion of the treatment, often a second remission is achieved. Celebrating this achievement atones for the hardship they have endured!

Coping with the unfortunate situation of cancer progression or recurrence after second-line treatment requires stamina and fortitude.

We must remember that cancer is a chronic disease. A third or even fourth line of treatment is still possible. Novel treatments are continuously developed and tested. They offer new hopes and buy quality time for patients who failed prior treatment. Clinical trials are used to test these novel approaches and frequently are validated for efficacy.

"Courage is not having the strength to go on, it is going on when you do not have strength."

Napoleon Bonaparte.

The past two decades witnessed great strides in cancer research. New discoveries and treatments are published every day. The successful deciphering of the genetic code of different cancer types opened new vistas in the understanding of the biology of cancer. Batches of new cancer drugs are regularly tested in the petri dish and lab animals, and many are found to be promising. To be able to bring the new agents from the lab bench to the clinic, one needs validation of safety and efficacy. To maintain objectivity and eliminate bias and subjectivity, stepwise clinical trials are designed. This ensures evidence-based, unbiased confirmation of the value of the new agent or treatment modality to qualify for FDA approval and certification (Federal Drug Administration).

What are the clinical trials? They are set up in three phases. Once a new agent or modality shows promise in lab tests, a phase-one clinical trial protocol is formulated. A limited number of patients who have exhausted all available standard treatments without success are offered the new experimental treatment on a voluntary basis. The purpose is to test the toxicity of the new agent and determine its "safe" dose. After the safe dose is determined, phase-two protocol is prepared to determine the efficacy of the new agent and its optimum dose. Phase three is a randomized trial protocol to compare the new treatment to a placebo (blank) or to an established treatment to determine with statistical certainty that the new treatment is both effective and safe compared to no treatment or superior to established treatment.

Clinical trials follow a strict compliance monitoring to ascertain high level of ethical standard and to avoid potential bias or misjudgment.

To this end, every clinical trial is listed on a government website, clinical trials.gov, to ensure transparency. The name and affiliation of the principal investigator and the trial registrar is stated. Cancer clinical trials are mostly proposed and administered by one of the major cancer research centers. However multi-institutional participation is open to qualified oncologists in community hospitals to widen the field of participation. Before a clinical trial protocol is launched, approval from an institutional review board is required. The board is composed of cancer specialists from different disciplines, the institute ethicist or chaplain, as well as a lay person from the community. The review board discusses the purpose, importance, and value of the proposal, and, above all, protecting the patient's dignity and their right for informed consent.

The clinical trials are financed by a variety of public and private grants. Among the public funds are National Institutes of Health, National Cancer Institute, Department of Defense, Medicare, and Veterans Administration. Among the private sponsors are American Cancer Society, pharmaceutical industry, and several other private and charity groups.

Patients enrolled in a clinical trial are selected based on defined criteria specified in the trial protocol. Once selected, the treating oncologist or oncology nurse would explain the purpose of the trial, what is being offered, the plan of treatment, the anticipated effects, and potential side effects. Patients and accompanying significant others would be offered the opportunity to ask questions and discuss any concerns. After the patient and accompanying person are satisfied with the information, an informed consent is signed. This is a document that states that the plan of treatment and potential side effects were explained and the patient with free will accepts the plan. The patient is then registered as enrolled in the trial, and the plan of treatment proceeds. Any follow-up exams and tests are periodically recorded in the file. The records are audited from time for timely completion. The principal investigator meets with the participating committee from time to time to monitor the progress of the trial and to report any deviation of the protocol to ensure the integrity of the records. Depending on the protocol specific length of evaluation, the number of enrollees required, and the target endpoint of the trial, the conclusion and evaluation will be made. The result, whether positive or negative, would then be reported to all the participants and eventually published in peer-reviewed scientific journals.

Patients may ask, Why would I participate in a clinical trial, and what is in it for me? This is a good question that should be addressed by the oncologist before signing the informed consent. If applicable, there are many advantages for participating in a clinical trial.

First, it gives access to a novel or new treatment agent that is otherwise not yet routinely available. Second, the new treatment may be expensive, and it would be provided free of charge for the trial participants. Third, all tests and exams during the trial are provided free of charge. Fourth, trial enrollees are keenly monitored and are subjected to extra attention and care. Lastly, participating in a clinical trial offers an opportunity to share in benefiting fellow patients who otherwise would not know the value of the novel treatment!

Confronted with recurrent or reactivated cancer, it is worthwhile to consider enrolling in a clinical trial. This offers a fresh possibility for trying a novel agent that otherwise is not available. It also renews hope for achieving a remission or at least stop the progression of the cancer.

Hope is eternal. A clinical trial at the end of the road is an incentive to pluck one's strength and brave the day!

CHAPTER EIGHT:

Acceptance...

"Cancer is a word, not a sentence."

John Diamond

The diagnosis of advanced stage cancer presents a challenge both to the patient as well as to the oncologist. The task of the oncologist is to gently present the problem as well as the solution. The emotional impact on the patient and family should not be underestimated. Explaining the difference between a serious and a hopeless situation is important.

Effectively managed advanced stage cancer can result in a long, comfortable life. The wisdom is to do our best, hope for the best, but to accept the outcome.

Fear and negligence are the most common barriers to early diagnosis. They result in denial or overlooking warning signs.

Realizing the seriousness of advanced stage cancer may lead the patient to feel a sense of guilt. It is therefore important to ease that feeling to overcome its negativity. Talking about the prognosis in cold, statistical numbers serves no purpose. What is relevant is the incentive to undergo effective treatment in terms of getting better by containing the progress of the disease. The response to the treatment would vary from person to person and from one type of cancer to another. But the objective is similar: to stop progression, to reduce the bulk of the disease, and to achieve a comfortable life, as long as possible.

In treating advanced stage cancer, chemotherapy and immunotherapy play an important part. This is because of the nature of advanced stage cancer involving local, regional, and distant spread, requiring a systemic approach to control the disease. After a remission is achieved, consolidation radiation treatments or even local surgery may be needed.

This rigorous treatment needs acceptance by the patient and family as it proceeds from cycle to cycle. To be able to cope, the need for supportive and symptomatic treatment should be addressed.

Although cure may not be achieved, improvement and longer survival are attainable. Changes in treatment with addition or substitution of one or more drug are proposed as the response, and toxicity is monitored. With the availability of new pharmaceutical agents, consideration for enrolling in a clinical trial may be proposed.

Going through the phases of the treatment, many patients find purpose in enduring the inconvenience and the side effects as they sail with hope and stamina. Parents may look forward to witnessing the graduation of their children. Grandparents may await the birth of a grandchild or the wedding of another. Having a purpose can miraculously provide strength and motivation.

CHAPTER NINE:
Approaching the End-Zone

"Get busy living or get busy dying."
Stephen King

Many cancer patients will be declared "cured." Others will survive with their cancer. The latter will go through treatments, and most of them will achieve remission. Some will experience a recurrence and reactivation of the cancer. They will be offered more treatment and perhaps will improve. Until such a point in time when cancer triumphs over available treatments. The clock will continue ticking, the heart continues beating, and the lungs continue breathing.

But the thoughts can be cloudy. That is when one's attitude can make the difference between joy and gloom. It may sound difficult in the beginning, but positive thinking and an optimistic attitude would make life worth living to the fullest. Add to this a measure of realism and acceptance. One golden rule: never ask your oncologist, "How long do I have left?" First, no one can give you a reliable answer, not even your oncologist. He or she can only give you a statistical range, which, when applied to an individual, is meaningless. Second, the question by itself implies a negative attitude. Though the news may not be cheerful, they do not have to be threatening. It may be helpful to remember how some celebrities handled their confrontation with incurable cancer.

Steve Jobs, founder of Apple, survived eight years after he was diagnosed with advanced cancer. In a speech he recounted his encounter with cancer as follows:

About a year ago I was diagnosed with cancer. I had a scan at 7:30 in the morning and it clearly showed a tumor on my pancreas. I did not even know what a pancreas was. The doctors told me this was almost certainly a type of cancer and that it is incurable and that I should expect to live no longer than three to six months. My doctor advised me to go home and get my affairs in order, which is doctor's code for prepare to die. It means to try to tell your kids everything you thought you would have the next ten years to tell them in just few months. It means to make sure everything is buttoned up so that it will be as easy as possible for your family. It means to say your goodbyes... This was the closest I have been to facing death... Having lived through it, I can now say this to you with a bit more certainty than when death was a useful but purely intellectual concept: No one wants to die. Even people who want to go to heaven do not want to die to get there. And yet death is the destination we all share. No one has ever escaped it. And that is as it should be, because death is likely the single best invention of life. It is life's change agent. It clears the old to make way for the new.

Steve Jobs survived with cancer several useful years after this speech.

Another celebrity: Ruth Bader Ginsburg, the second woman ever appointed to the Supreme Court. She was diagnosed with three different types of cancer over twenty years. Till the last day of her life, she continued to stay and work as a Supreme Court judge.

On an interview on *CBS This Morning* broadcast on September 29, 2019, Olivia Newton-John, the famous singer and performer, explained how to find joy in life with cancer. After she was treated for cancer of the breast and declared cancer free, she learned that the cancer has spread to her spine. She then received second-line treatment and went into remission. A few years later, the cancer recurred. She was disappointed but decided not to be angry. Instead, she decided to live her life from day to day. She pursued a purpose to help other human beings and that helped her cope with living with cancer.

Alex Trebek, a seven-time Emmy award winner for his popular TV program *Jeopardy*, was diagnosed with advanced pancreatic cancer on March 6, 2019, and continued to work on *Jeopardy* throughout his treatment. In March 2020, he announced that he had survived one year of cancer treatment, although he was told that he had only an 18 percent chance to live that long! He passed away on November 8, 2020.

The celebrities' examples mentioned above are a guide on how to handle the situation of facing the diagnosis of incurable cancer with a positive attitude. Instead of asking your oncologist what my prognosis is or how long I have to live, ask what can be done to make my survival comfortable and productive. If an investigational treatment or a clinical trial is suggested, ask what the objective of such treatment is and how would it impact your quality of life. The choice is yours based on informed expectation. Remember, there are always supportive treatments. These include pain control, nutritional supplements, physical therapy, and motivational help.

During this phase of life, a sober plan that fits your individual situation and needs would be prudent:

- Stay engaged in your current activity if you are able, and you find it fulfilling.
- Seek counsel from your spouse, partner, and family.
- Prepare or update your will and advance directives.
- Set your financial interests in order.
- Make a bucket list of things you wish to do and places you want to visit.
- Make peace with yourself and your acquaintances.
- Gather mementos of your life achievements that you wish to be remembered for. It would be meaningful to your family and friends.
- Ask your oncologist for information on hospice care.

At this point it may be appropriate to explain what hospice care is.

According to Hospice Foundation of America hospice is defined as:

- Medical care to help someone with terminal illness live as well as possible for as long as possible, increasing the quality of life.
- An interdisciplinary team of professionals who addresses physical, psychological, and spiritual distress focused on both the dying person and their entire family.
- Care that addresses symptom management, coordination of care, communication and decision making, clarification of goals of care, and quality of life.

The decision to enroll for hospice care should be discussed with patient and family and guided by the treating physician and hospice physician. It is usually considered when the patient's life expectation is six months or less, or that patient's health is rapidly deteriorating despite medical care, and the patient is ready to accept foregoing treatment that aims at prolonging life and instead wishes to live comfortably.

Medicare and Medicaid usually cover hospice care services, which include home visits by a physician, nurse, social worker, home-health aide, and spiritual counselor. Symptomatic and pain medications are also covered, as well as physical therapy and dietary counseling. If needed short, inpatient or respite care is provided, as well as grief counseling for patients and loved ones.

The last stage of one's life is better served with serenity and peace. Cancer being a chronic disease, death from cancer is not a surprise. Approaching the end zone takes time to reflect and prepare. This brings a sense of relief and fulfillment.

CHAPTER TEN:
Surviving Death!

*"When we are dead, seek not our tomb in the earth
but find it in the heart of people."*
Epitaph of Jalaludin Al Rumi

The intriguing title of this chapter may sound absurd and contradictory. But it should not be.

Let me explain. Life and death are a continuum of a cycle. Survival is living the present, for life is not forever. When we die, our memory survives. Our achievements, or lack thereof, remain and influence others. That is survival!

Dying of or with cancer is a journey. The journey is a process that starts with what is called the end-of-life. Death is the product. Its content is physiologic, emotional, and spiritual. Grievance and bereavement are the consumption of its value. This value can be sadness, relief, or growth. Dying as a process may be planned, improvised, or just a surprise, be it pleasant or unpleasant. Ideally, it should be planned. The plan may include personal preference and choice above and beyond a living will. This would depend on individual needs, availability, and circumstances. It could include receiving care at home, versus at a medical institution. The extent of end-of-life treatment may be just supportive, for the relief of symptoms and discomfort, or active, with additional cancer-specific treatments that may prolong life but may impact its quality.

During this period, the role of care givers and their interactions with the person they are caring for is important and requires thought, stamina, and endurance. To avoid stressful situations of exhaustion, resentment, disappointment, or even outright anger, wisdom and tact are needed. Attention to the mindset of the person cared for is important. Overprotection can sometimes be interpreted as total control or loss of autonomy and identity that results in resentment.

On the other hand, the caregiver can feel that the person they care for is too dependent and demanding. Either way, it is a situation to be avoided to create an atmosphere of respect and tranquility and to avoid later feelings of guilt and regret.

Though, death is a sad event because it is a loss of a life, of a needed support, of a friendship, or of a talent. Yet it can be grief mixed with relief. Relief that there is no more agonizing suffering. It is natural that one mourns the loss of a dear and near person. That is the human emotion of empathy and sympathy. But excessive and prolonged mourning is exhausting and depressive. It must be channeled into a positive energy. Instead of prolonged mourning, it can be a celebration of a life's achievement and pleasant shared memories. Healthy grieving is a release of the pain of loss. But prolonged mourning saps one's energy by prolonging the pain. A philosophical approach to life lightens the burden of grief. A spiritual approach also helps.

Since the dawn of human consciousness, death has baffled humanity. It was both accepted and denied. Funerals were ritualized to help the acceptance. The concept of afterlife was devised to deny the finality of death. Ancient Egyptians built pyramids to house the departed with provisions for their afterlife resurrection. Buddhism espoused the concept of resurrection in the sense of life recycling. Abrahamic religions promised heaven's paradise to reward the faithful or hell's dwelling afterlife for the sinners. Whatever the belief is, the human mind tries to take comfort in dealing with the predicament of death.

Realistically, everyone knows that life is not eternal. Surviving is living the present. Humans therefore must deal with this fact in such a way that brings peace to their minds.

Philosophically, one can accept death and deal with it as a fact of life. Alternatively, one can think about it spiritually whether through religious faith or esoteric mental connection. Spirituality connects our soul to a divine being that infuses our soul with an external energy. It gives purpose to our predicament, if not to help us cope with our grief but at least accept it.

Everyone has a unique way of grief. Some wish to talk about it. Some have different and changing levels of feelings. This emotional uncertainty can be exhausting and, if prolonged, may impact one's physical limits. It may lead to bouts of emotional upheavals and intense grief or even a sense of guilt. Spirituality and religious rituals can be of calming help, as they may give a meaning to the loss and offer peace to the troubled soul. Both remembrance and forgetfulness, in time, would help ease the grief. Treasured memories will remain, and the pain gradually heals.

Let us remember that life is the will to live. When the will to live surrenders, death becomes a peaceful fulfillment!

CHAPTER ELEVEN:
Looking Ahead

> *"Last fall I was diagnosed with stomach cancer.*
> *I've spent the last 6 months receiving chemo, radia-*
> *tion, and surgery. So far, so good. I need time to*
> *breathe, recover and relax.*
>
> *I am looking forward to spending this time with my*
> *family. But I will see fans sooner than later. I can't wait."*
> *A tweet by Toby Keith, Country Singer.*

Our desires and expectations are projected on our future. To fulfil our wishes and achieve our expectations, we must translate hope into action and act with determination.

Progress happens in sustainable increments. Thus, the invention of the microscope in 1590 paved the way for knowing the structure and function of the living cell. Studying the nucleus of the living cell led to understanding the mechanism of cell division and how the cancer cell, through its genetic material, multiplies. That genetic material contained in the DNA of the cell carries the instructions and information that the cell needs for its growth and reproduction.

In the span of many years, several researchers added increments of knowledge about the nature and significance of the living cell DNA.

In 1953 James Watson and Francis Crick discovered the structure of DNA molecule as a double helix formed of a spiraling intertwined structure. Detailed knowledge of human DNA is of great importance for research on cancer. The DNA of the living cell contains the "program" that determines the cell characteristics and its behavior. Beginning on October 1, 1990, an international research team embarked on mapping the molecular DNA makeup of the entire human genome, meaning all the genes of human beings, under the banner The Human Genome Project. With contributions from international researchers throughout the USA, UK, France, Germany, Japan, and China, the project was completed in April 2003. This achievement meant that the inner secret of human DNA was unlocked. Vital information that passes from generation to generation of human cells can now be accessible for cancer researchers to study the mechanisms that cause a normal cell to transform into a cancer cell. This knowledge would help identify persons who inherit certain alterations in their genes that make them susceptible to develop certain diseases or predisposes them to have cancer.

Cancer researchers would also be able to explore gene therapy for prevention or discover new therapeutic agents for treatment.

Another milestone in the quest for cancer cure is the "Cancer Moonshot Project." In December 2016 the US Congress passed the 21st Century Cures Act, authorizing $1.8 billion in funding over seven years. The goals are to reduce the death from cancer by at least 50 percent over the next twenty-five years and improve the experience of people and their families living with and surviving cancer.

Thus, looking forward, cancer researchers are excited about the tremendous possibilities opened to harness modern technology and the accumulated database to be able to identify persons who are at risk to develop cancer. It may be possible to avert the risk by correcting a genetic aberration. Early diagnosis through a simple blood test is becoming available in certain cases. More effective evidence-based treatments discovered in the lab are gradually becoming available at the bedside through well-designed clinical trials. Personalized treatments based on individual characteristics of the cancer is now available as investigational, but in the future, it may be technically streamlined so that it becomes more affordable.

Today's cancer survival wishes shall be the promise of tomorrow!

SOURCES FOR ADDITIONAL TRUSTED INFORMATION

"Trust but verify"

Ronald Reagan.

National Cancer Institute, Comprehensive Cancer Information: https://www.cancer.gov

American Cancer Society: https://www.Cancer.org

US Administration on Aging: https://www.eldercare.gov

Hospice care: https://www.hospicefoundation.org

United States Cancer Statistics: https://cdc.gov >cancer >uscs

National Comprehensive Cancer Network. (NCCN):
www.nccn.org

ACKNOWLEDGMENTS

A word of thanks to Barbara, my wife, for persuading me to structure my retirement time so I penned this narrative.

I also appreciate the willingness of Dr. Donna M. Powell, Senior Scientist, NCCN, to read my first draft and for her valued comments.

My endless gratitude goes to my patients, who, over the years of my professional life, have taught me the meaning of survival.